STUDY GUIDE ON PRAYER

by
Shirley Crowder

N

Pix-N-Pens
Publishing

Study Guide On Prayer
© 2017 Shirley Crowder

ISBN-13: 978-1-944120-27-6
ISBN-10: 1-944120-27-0
Ebook ISBN: 978-1-944120-28-3

Numerous quotes taken from *Prayer: It's Not About You* Copyright © 2016 by Harriet E Michael; Pix-N-Pens Publishing. Used by permission. All rights reserved worldwide.

Scriptures are taken from the Holy Bible, New International Version®, NIV®. Copyright © 1973, 1978, 1984, 2011 by Biblica, Inc.™ Used by permission of Zondervan. All rights reserved worldwide. www.zondervan.com.

Published by:
Pix-N-Pens Publishing
PO Box 702852
Dallas, TX 75370
www.PixNPens.com

COMPANION TO

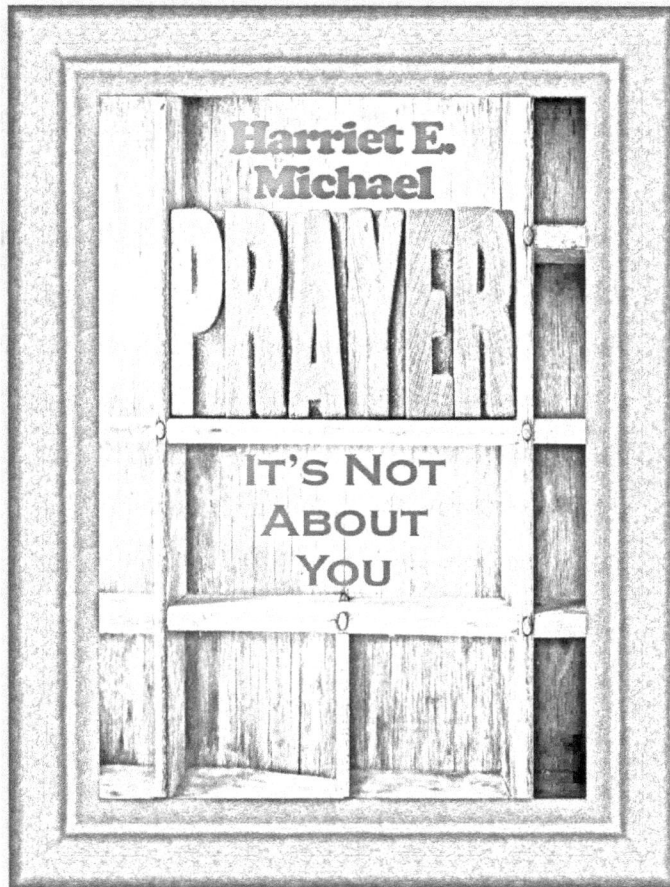

**Available on Kindle and in paperback
from Amazon.**

PREFACE

As soon as Shirley received her copy of **Prayer: It's Not About You**, she began marking it and thinking about how to teach the book to a group of ladies. This study guide is the compilation of the reading and homework assignments this group worked through. She appreciates these ladies for their invaluable help fine-tuning this study guide.

With appreciation for the provision of God's grace, she thanks the myriad of men and women who have taught and shown her how to pray, and to study God's Word.

It has been a joy for her to work with her lifelong best friend, Harriet Michael, who authored the original text of **Prayer: It's Not About You.**

She thanks her publisher, Marji Laine Clubine, who has advised and encouraged her throughout the process of bringing this study guide to publication.

What an honor for her to work with her MK (missionary kid) cousin, Baker Hill, who prioritized her request to review the manuscript and apply his expertise to improve and refine the content, accuracy, and consistency of her words.

TABLE OF CONTENTS

INTRODUCTION

God created us as relational creatures who are to reflect His glory to a world that is lost and dying without hope. Think about your earthly relationships. Once you met a person, how did you get to know him or her? The two of you spent time together and got to know each other, right? One of you listened while the other talked, and vice versa.

Christ-followers have received God's gracious gift of salvation that brings us into relationship with Him. We cultivate our relationship with God by spending time listening to Him and talking to Him. God's primary way of speaking to us today is through the Holy Spirit-inspired Bible. Our way of speaking to God is through prayer. Our ability to trust God as we pray is directly related to how intimately we know God as our Savior, Creator, Father, and Lord.

As you work your way through this study guide, you will read *Prayer: It's Not About You*, chapter by chapter. Then you will be guided to interact with the teachings, principles, and practices contained in Scripture and *Prayer: It's Not About You*.

It is the author's prayer that as you work through this *Study Guide on Prayer*, you will gain knowledge and a better understanding of prayer. This knowledge and understanding, through the work of the Holy Spirit, will lead you to incorporate the teachings, principles, and practices in Scripture and the book into your prayer life so that as your passion to pray increases, resulting in a strengthened relationship with God the Father through Jesus Christ His Son.

HOW TO USE THIS GUIDE

FOR INDIVIDUAL STUDY

For each chapter, you will be led to:

➤ **PRAY,** asking the Lord to open the eyes of your heart so that you learn what you need to know about prayer and that you would be sensitive to the Holy Spirit's conviction of sin, prompting you toward change. As the Holy Spirit convicts you of sin, stop and ask forgiveness for that sin and for strength to choose not to continue practicing that sin.

➤ **READ** a chapter in *Prayer: It's Not About You.* As you read the chapter, take time to look up each Scripture passage in your Bible, noting the context of the passage within the chapter and book of the Bible in which it is found. In the space provided, you will record at least two teachings, principles, and/or practices that stand out to you. And, you will record any questions, teachings, principles, and/or practices you need to study further.

➤ **DIG DEEPER** into the teachings, principles, and practices by prayerfully considering your responses, explanations, and descriptions. Here you will also take time to research and further study the questions, teachings, principles, and/or practices you recorded in the previous section. Using your Bible, commentaries, and other resources (print or online), you will research and study these questions, teachings, principles, and/or practices, making note of your answers and what you have learned from your research and study.

➤ **SCRIPTURE EMPHASIS** leads you to carefully read and meditate upon a Scripture passage. You will record teachings, principles, and practices from the passage, and answer questions that the Holy Spirit will help you know how to integrate into your Christian walk.

➤ **QUESTIONS FOR REFLECTION** are the same, with a few exceptions, as those found on the last page of each chapter in the book. Prayerfully consider your answers, thoughts, and emotions, and record them in the space provided.

- ➤ **NOW WHAT?** allows you time to interact with what you have learned about prayer, and evaluate specific teachings, principles, and/or practices you need to incorporate into your prayer life.

- ➤ **APPLY WHAT YOU LEARNED** by praying according to that particular chapter's teachings, principles, and practices, and asking the Lord to help you incorporate the teachings, principles, and practices into your prayer life.

- ➤ **MORE ANSWERS, NOTES, THOUGHTS, AND QUESTIONS** provides extra space for answers that may not fit in the space provided within the study guide. Here you may also record any answers, notes, thoughts, and questions that you have not yet answered.

WRAP-UP (after Chapter 14: "Conclusion") will lead you to:

- ➤ **REVIEW** the teachings, principles, and/or practices in each chapter of the study guide.

- ➤ **LIST** from each chapter of the study guide any teachings, principles, and/or practices of which you still do not have a good understanding. Also, list questions that remain unanswered after your research and study.

- ➤ **PERSIST** until you have researched and studied each teaching, principle, and/or practice listed above and you have a good understanding of each one.

- ➤ **ANSWER** the questions from the "List" section using your research and study from the "Persist" section. Explain the answers as you would to a new Christ-follower.

EVEN MORE ANSWERS, NOTES, THOUGHTS, AND QUESTIONS

Here you will find additional space for answers that may not have fit in the space provided within the study guide chapters. You may also record any answers, notes, thoughts, and questions that you have not yet answered.

📖 **indicates either a direct quote from *Prayer: It's Not About You*
or directs you to read a specific portion of the book.**

FOR SMALL GROUPS

GROUP LEADER

For each chapter, you will be led to:

➢ **COMPLETE** each chapter's reading and study assignments (see study guide pp. 9-10 "For Individual Study").

As you work through the week's study guide chapter:

➢ **ANTICIPATE** teachings, principles, and practices that may be difficult for some of the group members to understand and accept, and be prepared to explain them.

➢ **BEGIN** the discussion on time.

➢ **FACILITATE** a structured discussion using the study guide components as your outline.

➢ **ENSURE** the discussion stays on track and no one person dominates the discussion time.

➢ **MONITOR** the discussion so it is based on biblical truth, not the feelings and/or opinions of group members.

➢ **ENGAGE** the entire group in the discussion.

➢ **ENCOURAGE** group members to complete the reading and study assignments each week.

➢ **CONCLUDE** the discussion and end on time.

GROUP MEMBERS

For each chapter, you will be led to:

➢ **COMPLETE** each chapter's reading and study assignments (see study guide pp. 9-10 "For Individual Study").

CHAPTER 1: WHY PRAY?

➤ **PRAY,** asking the Lord to open the eyes of your heart to learn what you need to know about prayer and that you would be sensitive to the Holy Spirit's conviction of sin, prompting you toward change. As the Holy Spirit convicts you of sin in your life, stop and ask forgiveness for that sin and for strength to choose not to continue practicing that sin.

➤ **READ** Chapter 1: "Why Pray?" in *Prayer: It's Not About You.*

List at least two of the teachings, principles, and/or practices that stood out to you as you read this chapter.

What difference would it make if you incorporated these teachings, principles, and/or practices into your prayer life?

What questions, teachings, principles, and/or practices do you need to research and study further?

➤ **DIG DEEPER** into the following teachings, principles, and practices by prayerfully considering your responses, explanations, and descriptions. Record them in the space provided.

📖 **"At times prayer is agonizing because it increases my awareness of the pain or ugliness of a situation."** (pp. 3-4)
Briefly describe a time when prayer was agonizing for you as it increased your awareness of the pain and ugliness of the situation about which you were praying.

What did you learn about God and prayer during this time?

📖 **"... prayer is a mighty weapon in the hands of a believer who understands and uses it correctly."** (p. 4)
Tell of a time you have experienced or witnessed the result of the mighty weapon of prayer.

What did you learn about God and prayer during this time?

Review the seven conclusions listed on pages 6-7 of *Prayer: It's Not About You*. Explain how each of these conclusions compel you to pray.

📖 1) **God commands us to pray.**

📖 2) **Prayer is important.**

📖 3) **Prayer does not change God's plan, rather it helps to bring that plan into action.**

📖 4) **Prayer has value.**

📖 5) **We need to be tenacious in our prayers.**

📖 6) **God answers prayers.**

📖 7) **We should be prepared for how prayer will affect our lives.**

STUDY GUIDE ON PRAYER

📖 **"My understanding of prayer has also been shaped through personal experiences."** (p. 7)

Describe how personal experiences have shaped your understanding of prayer?

Take time now to research and further study the questions, teachings, principles, and/or practices you recorded in the "Read" section of this chapter's study guide. Use your Bible, commentaries, and other resources (print or online) to study these questions, teachings, principles, and/or practices. Make notes of your answers and what you have learned from your research and study.

➢ **SCRIPTURE EMPHASIS**

Carefully read and meditate upon Ephesians 6:13-20. Write your answers to the following in the space provided.

How does prayer relate to the whole armor of God?

What application does this passage have for your prayer life?

What questions do you have about this passage that are not addressed in the book?

Use your Bible, commentaries, and other resources (print or online) to find biblical answers for your questions, and record them below.

➤ **QUESTIONS FOR REFLECTION**
Prayerfully consider your answers, thoughts, and emotions. Record them in the space provided.

📖 **Does prayer have any real power?** Explain.

📖 **Does prayer change God's plan or does it change the people and circumstances around us to accord with God's plan?** Record Scripture references in explaining your answer.

📖 **Do our prayers provoke God to act on our behalf in accordance with His great plan? (Did God act before, after, or *as* Elijah prayed?)** Defend your answer using Scripture.

📖 **How did other prayer warriors in the Bible pray?**

📖 **Are there any common threads running through all the prayers of these prayer warriors?** (See previous question.)

➤ **NOW WHAT?**

Based on your study of the "Why Pray?" chapter, what specific teachings, principles, and/or practices do you need to incorporate into your prayer life? Record them below.

➢ **APPLY WHAT YOU LEARNED** by asking the Lord to help you become a mighty prayer warrior. Thank Him for the prayer warriors who have prayed for you throughout your life. Ask Him to enable you to incorporate into your prayer life the teachings, principles, and/or practices you recorded earlier in the "Now What?" section of this chapter's study guide. Make notes of specific things for which you should pray.

➤ **More Answers, Notes, Thoughts, and Questions**

OLD TESTAMENT

📖 *"We have taken a wartime walkie-talkie*
and tried to turn it into a civilian intercom
to call the servants for another cushion in the den."

John Piper in *Desiring God*

CHAPTER 2: MOSES

➤ **PRAY,** asking the Lord to open the eyes of your heart to learn what you need to know about prayer and that you would be sensitive to the Holy Spirit's conviction of sin, prompting you toward change. As the Holy Spirit convicts you of sin in your life, stop and ask forgiveness for that sin and for strength to choose not to continue practicing that sin.

➤ **READ** Chapter 2: "Moses" in *Prayer: It's Not About You.*

List at least two of the teachings, principles, and/or practices that stood out to you as you read this chapter.

What difference would it make if you incorporated these teachings, principles, and/or practices into your prayer life?

What questions, teachings, principles, and/or practices do you need to research and study further?

➤ **DIG DEEPER** into the following teachings, principles, and practices by prayerfully considering your responses, explanations, and descriptions. Record them in the space provided.

📖 **"God wants us to be completely dependent on Him, not on ourselves."** (p. 16)

In what ways have you been prone to depend upon yourself and not God?

📖 Review the three levels of struggle on page 17.

Think of a situation through which you have struggled and briefly describe it in terms of the three levels of struggle, making sure to include your thoughts, emotions, and reactions.

1. The battle that was raging (spiritually, emotionally, mentally, and physically).

2. The intercessor who lifted his or her hands toward God and asked God for help in the battle.

3. The men and women who came alongside you, and the specific practical ways they helped you.

What did you learn about God and prayer during this situation?

📖 **"It is important to note that the people were not repentant. They had not asked Moses to intercede for them, but he did anyway because he was burdened by their sin."** (p. 20)
Who are the unrepentant people in your life for whom you have interceded?

Who are the unrepentant people in your life for whom are you not interceding?

Create and record a plan for how you will intercede for the unrepentant people in your life.

📖 **"Some points from this interaction between God and Moses can be applied to our own prayers of intercession."** (p. 21)
Describe how you have applied each of the following to your own prayers of intercession.

📖 **"Love the Lord your God with all your heart and with all your soul and with all your mind."** (p. 22)

📖 **"Love your neighbor as yourself."** (p. 23)

📖 **"He (Moses) petitioned God based on God Himself."** (p. 23)

📖 **"He (Moses) petitioned God numerous times with the same request."** (p. 23)

📖 On pages 28 and 29 of *Prayer: It's Not About Me* we read the account of Moses not being allowed to enter the land for which he had searched most of his life.

Think of a situation in which the Lord did not allow you to do something or get something you wanted. Briefly describe that situation, and record your thoughts, emotions, and reactions.

Take time now to research and further study the questions, teachings, principles, and/or practices you recorded in the "Read" section of this chapter's study guide. Use your Bible, commentaries, and other resources (print or online) to study these questions, teachings, principles, and/or practices. Make notes of your answers and what you have learned from your research and study.

➢ **SCRIPTURE EMPHASIS**
Carefully read and meditate upon Numbers 12:1-3. Write your answers to the following in the space provided.

What do we learn about Moses from this passage?

What application does this passage have for your prayer life?

What questions do you have about this passage that are not addressed in the book?

Use your Bible, commentaries, and other resources (print or online) to find biblical answers for your questions, and record them below.

➢ **QUESTIONS FOR REFLECTION**

Prayerfully consider your answers, thoughts, and emotions. Record them in the space provided.

📖 **Why did God choose Moses to be the intercessor for His people?**

📖 **What two commandments did Moses exemplify?**

📖 **Moses often doubted how God would do something and sometimes even argued with God, but what proved how much he loved God?**

📖 **What can we learn about being a prayer warrior from Moses?**

➤ **NOW WHAT?**
Based on your study of the "Moses" chapter, what specific teachings, principles, and/or practices do you need to incorporate into your prayer life?

➤ **APPLY WHAT YOU LEARNED** by asking the Lord to give you wisdom and discernment in how to intercede for those whom He has placed in your life. Thank Him for all those who have interceded for you throughout your life. Ask Him to enable you to incorporate into your prayer life the teachings, principles, and/or practices you recorded earlier in the "Now What?" section of this chapter's study guide. Make notes of specific things for which you should pray.

> ➤ **MORE ANSWERS, NOTES, THOUGHTS, AND QUESTIONS**

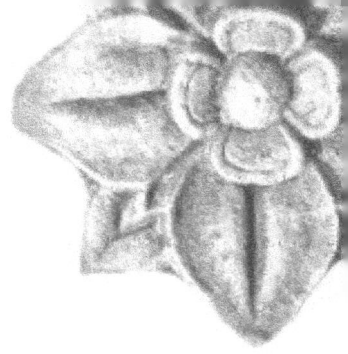

CHAPTER 3: DAVID / THE PSALMS — PART 1

➤ **PRAY,** asking the Lord to open the eyes of your heart to learn what you need to know about prayer and that you would be sensitive to the Holy Spirit's conviction of sin, prompting you toward change. As the Holy Spirit convicts you of sin in your life, stop and ask forgiveness for that sin and for strength to choose not to continue practicing that sin.

➤ **READ** through the end of #3 on page 43 of Chapter 3: "David / the Psalms" in *Prayer: It's Not About You.*

List at least two teachings, principles, and/or practices that stood out to you as you read this chapter.

What difference would it make if you incorporated these teachings, principles, and/or practices into your prayer life?

What questions, teachings, principles, and/or practices do you need to research and study further?

➤ **DIG DEEPER** into the following teachings, principles, and practices by prayerfully considering your responses, explanations, and descriptions. Record them in the space provided.

David

📖 **"God's plans are not our plans. They often do not fit our ideas of how things should go."** (p. 31)

Tell about a time in your life when God's plans were not your plans.

Describe how you reacted, making sure to include your thoughts, emotions, and reactions.

📖 **"What seems confusing to Christians is the idea that God would bring about brokenness and pain in a person's life through the person's own failures or even sins ..."** (p. 32)

When has God brought about brokenness and pain in your life through your own failures and/or sin?

STUDY GUIDE ON PRAYER

Describe how you reacted, making sure to include your thoughts, emotions, and reactions.

📖 **"… anytime we pray in an attempt to get God to work according to our agenda, however benevolent that agenda may seem, instead of surrendering our will to His, we are praying amiss."** (p. 35)
Recall and summarize a time you prayed amiss about something.

How did you realize you were praying amiss?

What did you learn as a result of praying amiss?

The Psalms

📖 Review #1 – #3 of the ten themes or points of prayer on pages 38-43. Explain how each of the following themes or points does or does not impact your prayer life.

📖 **1) Prayers are addressed to, or directed toward God, the Father.**

📖 **2) Prayers contain praise and thanksgiving.**

📖 **3) We should confess our sins and recognize our personal unworthiness.**

Take time now to research and further study the questions, teachings, principles, and/or practices you recorded in the "Read" section of this chapter's study guide. Use your Bible, commentaries, and other resources (print or online) to study these questions, teachings, principles, and/or practices. Make notes of your answers and what you have learned from your research and study.

➢ **SCRIPTURE EMPHASIS**

Carefully read and meditate upon 2 Samuel 12:16-23. Write your answers to the following in the space provided.

What does this passage teach us about God answering our prayers in ways we do not desire?

How are Christ-followers to respond when God answers our prayers in ways we do not desire?

What questions do you have about this passage that are not addressed in the book?

Use your Bible, commentaries, and other resources (print or online) to find biblical answers for your questions, and record them below.

➢ QUESTIONS FOR REFLECTION

Prayerfully consider your answers, thoughts, and emotions. Record them in the space provided.

📖 **What does it mean to pray amiss?**

📖 **When did David pray amiss?**

STUDY GUIDE ON PRAYER

What kind of man or woman does God choose for His work?

➢ **NOW WHAT?**
Based on your study of the "David" portion of "David / the Psalms" chapter, what specific teachings, principles, and/or practices do you need to incorporate into your prayer life? Record them below.

➢ **APPLY WHAT YOU LEARNED** by asking the Lord to give you a heart that is quick to repent when confronted with sin. Ask Him to enable you to trust Him enough to pray according to His will, and to transform your will into His will. Ask Him to enable you to incorporate into your prayer life the teachings, principles, and/or practices you recorded earlier in the "Now What?" section of this chapter's study guide. Make notes of specific things for which you should pray.

➤ **MORE ANSWERS, NOTES, THOUGHTS, AND QUESTIONS**

STUDY GUIDE ON PRAYER

CHAPTER 3: DAVID / THE PSALMS — PART 2

➤ **PRAY,** asking the Lord to open the eyes of your heart to learn what you need to know about prayer and that you would be sensitive to the Holy Spirit's conviction of sin, prompting you toward change. As the Holy Spirit convicts you of sin in your life, stop and ask forgiveness for that sin and for strength to choose not to continue practicing that sin.

➤ **READ** beginning with #4 on page 43 of Chapter 3: "David / the Psalms" in *Prayer: It's Not About You.*

List at least two teachings, principles, and/or practices that stood out to you as you read this passage.

What difference would it make if you incorporated these teachings, principles, and/or practices into your prayer life?

What questions, teachings, principles, and/or practices do you need to research and study further?

➢ **DIG DEEPER** into the following teachings, principles, and practices by prayerfully considering your responses, explanations, and descriptions. Record them in the space provided.

The Psalms

📖 Review #4 – #10 of the ten themes or points of prayer. (pp. 43-60)
Explain how each of the following themes or points does or does not impact your prayer life.

📖 **4) We can petition God based on His character.**

📖 **God's steadfast love**

📖 **Faithfulness**

📖 **Fortress / Stronghold / Rock / Refuge**

📖 **Shield**

📖 **Help**

📖 **Deliverer / Redeemer**

📖 **Goodness and Mercy**

📖 **Graciousness**

📖 **Righteous / Upright / Holy**

📖 **Other Character Traits**

📖 **5) We can petition God based on His promises.**

📖 **6) We can petition God based on His ability to answer our prayer—asking Him to just do it!**

📖 7) We can petition God based on His sovereign will.

📖 8) We can petition God based on His own glory—for the sake of His own glory or for the sake of His name.

📖 9) We should recognize what God has done in our lives—remembering His blessings and answered prayers, and thanking Him for them.

📖 10) We can pour out our hearts to God.

Take time now to research and further study the questions, teachings, principles, and/or practices you recorded in the "Read" section of this chapter's study guide. Use your Bible, commentaries, and other resources (print or online) to study these questions, teachings, principles, and/or practices. Make notes of your answers and what you have learned from your research and study.

➤ **SCRIPTURE EMPHASIS**
Carefully read and meditate upon Psalm 69:1-3. Write your answers to the following in the space provided.

What does this passage teach about God?

What does this passage teach about prayer?

What questions do you have about this passage that are not addressed in the book?

Use your Bible, commentaries, and other resources (print or online) to find biblical answers for your questions, and record them below.

> QUESTIONS FOR REFLECTION

Prayerfully consider your answers, thoughts, and emotions. Record them in the space provided.

📖 **Name the guidelines for the content of our prayers.**

Record some ways that you can keep your prayers God-focused rather than self-focused.

Briefly explain what effect unconfessed sin has on your ability to pray and the content of your prayers.

> **NOW WHAT?**
> Based on your study of "The Psalms" portion of "David / the Psalms" chapter, what specific teachings, principles, and/or practices do you need to incorporate into your prayer life? Record them below.

> **APPLY WHAT YOU LEARNED** by asking the Lord to give you a better understanding of His character so that you will trust Him in times when your prayers are not answered in the way you want them answered. Ask Him to teach you to worship Him when He answers your prayers differently than you want them answered. Ask Him to enable you to incorporate into your prayer life the teachings, principles, and/or practices you recorded earlier in the "Now What?" section of this chapter's study guide. Make notes of specific things for which you should pray.

➤ **More Answers, Notes, Thoughts, and Questions**

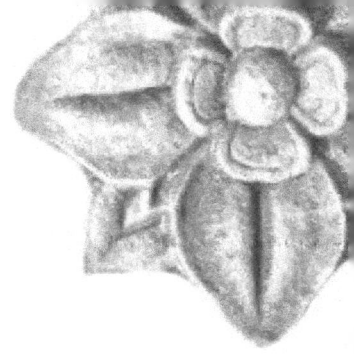

CHAPTER 4: HANNAH, SAMUEL, DANIEL, NEHEMIAH, EZRA, AND HABAKKUK

➤ **PRAY,** asking the Lord to open the eyes of your heart to learn what you need to know about prayer and that you would be sensitive to the Holy Spirit's conviction of sin, prompting you toward change. As the Holy Spirit convicts you of sin in your life, stop and ask forgiveness for that sin and for strength to choose not to continue practicing that sin.

➤ **READ** Chapter 4: "Hannah, Samuel, Daniel, Nehemiah, Ezra, and Habakkuk" in *Prayer: It's Not About You.*

List at least two of the teachings, principles, and/or practices that stood out to you as you read this chapter.

What difference would it make if you incorporated these teachings, principles, and/or practices into your prayer life?

What questions, teachings, principles, and/or practices do you need to research and study further?

➤ **DIG DEEPER** into the following teachings, principles, and practices by prayerfully considering your responses, explanations, and descriptions. Record them in the space provided.

📖 **Hannah: "She prayed earnestly for a child … Eli the priest thought she was drunk … she explained that she was not drunk, she was pouring her heart out to God because of her intense desire to have a child.** (p. 65)
How can you know whether the desire of your heart is from God and not from your own selfish desire or the evil one?

📖 **Samuel: "… we learn to obey God even when we do not like what He has told us to do."** (p. 71)
Think about a time when you obeyed God even though you did not like what His Word told you to do. What thoughts did you have, and what emotions did you experience during that time?

📖 **Daniel: "He studied Jeremiah's prophecy concerning Jerusalem and became aware of God's plan, causing him to turn to God in prayer to petition Him according to that plan."** (pp. 71-72)
Explain the importance of reading and studying God's Word in order to know His will and pray according to His will.

📖 **Nehemiah: "He had inquired as to the wellbeing of the Jews who had escaped and survived the exile, as well as the condition of the city of Jerusalem. He received discouraging news."** (p. 73)

How do you react when you hear distressing news?

How is your reaction to distressing news similar to or different from Nehemiah's?

📖 **Ezra:** On pages 76-77 we read that when Ezra heard God's people were deliberately disobeying Him by intermarrying, he tore his clothes, pulled out his hair and beard, and sat down appalled, because he understood the gravity of their sin.

Describe your understanding of sin.

Describe the difference in the sin of someone who lies to their boss about being sick and someone who molests a child.

📖 **Habakkuk: "But Habakkuk determined in his heart that he would accept from the hand of God whatever God brought, knowing that no matter how frightened he was, or how unpleasant the fulfillment of the vision might be, God would be acting according to His sovereign will." (p. 79)**
What would you say to a new Christ-follower about how you are able to determine something in your heart?

Record details of a situation in which you have determined in your heart to do something, and the result of your doing that thing.

Take time now to research and further study the questions, teachings, principles, and/or practices you recorded in the "Read" section of this chapter's study guide. Use your Bible, commentaries, and other resources (print or online) to study these questions, teachings, principles, and/or practices. Make notes of your answers and what you have learned from your research and study.

➢ **SCRIPTURE EMPHASIS**

Carefully read and meditate upon Habakkuk 3:3-15. Write your answers to the following in the space provided.

Why did Habakkuk include all of this history in his prayer?

Expound upon how the principle modeled here helps us know how and for what to pray.

What questions do you have about this passage that are not addressed in the book?

Use your Bible, commentaries, and other resources (print or online) to find biblical answers for your questions, and record them below.

➤ QUESTIONS FOR REFLECTION

Prayerfully consider your answers, thoughts, and emotions. Record them in the space provided.

📖 **What important lesson about prayer do we learn from Hannah?**

📖 **If our prayers are answered favorably, what does this indicate about our understanding of God's plan?**

📖 **What similarities can be drawn between the prayers of Daniel, Nehemiah, and Ezra, and the other prayers that we have seen so far in the book?**

📖 **What specifically did Daniel, Nehemiah, and Ezra do or say that indicated their earnestness as well as recognition of their needy state?**

📖 **What do we learn from Habakkuk's prayer?**

➤ **NOW WHAT?**

Based on your study of the "Hannah, Samuel, Daniel, Nehemiah, Ezra, and Habakkuk" chapter, what specific teachings, principles, and/or practices do you need to incorporate into your prayer life? Record them below.

➢ **APPLY WHAT YOU LEARNED** by asking the Lord to enable you to trust Him to develop the desires of your heart into His desires, and that you will come to know Him well enough to have faith to obey Him, even when you do not like what His Word tells you to do. Ask Him to enable you to incorporate into your prayer life the teachings, principles, and/or practices you recorded earlier in the "Now What?" section of this chapter's study guide. Make notes of specific things for which you should pray.

➤ **MORE ANSWERS, NOTES, THOUGHTS, AND QUESTIONS**

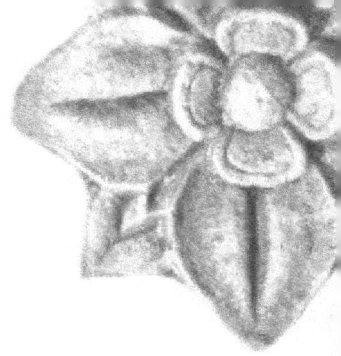

CHAPTER 5: ABRAHAM, JACOB, HEZEKIAH, SOLOMON, AND JEHOSHAPHAT

➤ **PRAY,** asking the Lord to open the eyes of your heart to learn what you need to know about prayer and that you would be sensitive to the Holy Spirit's conviction of sin, prompting you toward change. As the Holy Spirit convicts you of sin in your life, stop and ask forgiveness for that sin and for strength to choose not to continue practicing that sin.

➤ **READ** Chapter 5: "Abraham, Jacob, Hezekiah, Solomon, and Jehoshaphat" in *Prayer: It's Not About You.*

List at least two of the teachings, principles, and/or practices that stood out to you as you read this chapter.

What difference would it make if you incorporated these teachings, principles, and/or practices into your prayer life?

What questions, teachings, principles, and/or practices do you need to research and study further?

➢ **DIG DEEPER** into the following teachings, principles, and practices by prayerfully considering your responses, explanations, and descriptions. Record them in the space provided.

📖 **Abraham: "Yet in spite of his human frailties, Abraham boldly made his request to God. These requests were consistent with God's ability to protect His own. We also see from Abraham's prayer the practice of being persistent in our petitions, and the fact that God answers the prayers of His people."** (p. 85)
What principles of prayer do you see at work in this quote?

📖 **Jacob: "He feared for his life and for the lives of his family. Yet he was able to draw strength from his memory of God's promises to him."** (p. 85)
From which promises of God do you draw strength?

📖 **Hezekiah: "In this prayer** (Isaiah 37:16-20)**, Hezekiah's sole basis for asking God's help was the fact that God's name was at stake."** (p. 88)
Describe a situation when your reason for asking God's help was because His name was at stake. If you have never prayed on the basis that God's name was at stake, describe a situation that would lend itself to this type of praying.

📖 **Solomon: "In this prayer Solomon did not articulate as much personal humility or brokenness as we have seen in other prayers. Rather, he expressed the corporate humility of the people …."** (p. 92)

Give modern-day examples of times and places where it would be good for a leader to express to God the humility of his or her people.

📖 **Jehoshaphat: "There was a time when some armies came against Jehoshaphat intending to do battle with his armies. Afraid, Jehoshaphat set his face to seek the Lord."** (p. 92)

What does it mean to set your face to seek the Lord?

Tell of a time when you set your face to seek the Lord.

Take time now to research and further study the questions, teachings, principles, and/or practices you recorded in the "Read" section of this chapter's study guide. Use your Bible, commentaries, and other resources (print or online) to study these questions, teachings, principles, and/or practices. Make notes of your answers and what you have learned from your research and study.

> **SCRIPTURE EMPHASIS**

Carefully read and meditate upon II Chronicles 1:7-12. Write your answers to the following in the space provided.

Examine the things for which you most often pray and record them below.

How are the types of things for which you pray in line or not in line with the prayer principle found in this passage?

STUDY GUIDE ON PRAYER

What questions do you have about this passage that are not addressed in the book?

Use your Bible, commentaries, and other resources (print or online) to find biblical answers for your questions, and record them below.

➤ **QUESTIONS FOR REFLECTION**
Prayerfully consider your answers, thoughts, and emotions. Record them in the space provided.

📖 **What do Abraham's prayers teach us?**

📖 **What practical lesson do we learn from Abraham about dealing with challenging situations, times when we are discouraged and our faith is tested?**

📖 What effect did prayer have on Jacob and how does the late Adrian Rogers state this truth?

📖 Solomon's prayer for wisdom sheds light on the type of prayer that pleases God. What elements does a prayer that pleases God contain?

📖 In addition to praying for others, what else does Hezekiah's second prayer show it is appropriate to pray?

📖 What is particularly interesting about the timing of the people of Judah's praise in regard to Jehoshaphat's prayer?

➢ **NOW WHAT?**
Based on your study of the "Abraham, Jacob, Hezekiah, Solomon, and Jehoshaphat" chapter, what specific teachings, principles, and/or practices do you need to incorporate into your prayer life? Record them below.

➢ **APPLY WHAT YOU LEARNED** by asking the Lord to give you wisdom, and strengthen you to set your face to seek Him. Ask Him to enable you to know Him better so that you will trust His sovereign plan. Thank the Lord for the teachings, principles, and practices that you learned. Ask Him to enable you to incorporate into your prayer life the teachings, principles, and/or practices you recorded earlier in the "Now What?" section of this chapter's study guide. Make notes of specific things for which you should pray.

> ## MORE ANSWERS, NOTES, THOUGHTS, AND QUESTIONS

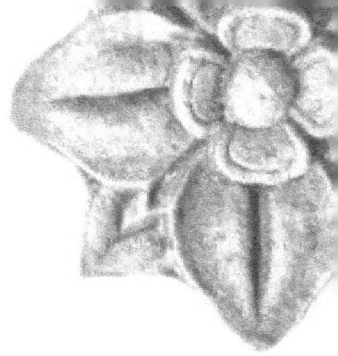

CHAPTER 6: JOB

➢ **PRAY,** asking the Lord to open the eyes of your heart to learn what you need to know about prayer and that you would be sensitive to the Holy Spirit's conviction of sin, prompting you toward change. As the Holy Spirit convicts you of sin in your life, stop and ask forgiveness for that sin and for strength to choose not to continue practicing that sin.

➢ **READ** Chapter 6: "Job" in *Prayer: It's Not About You.*

List at least two of the teachings, principles, and/or practices that stood out to you as you read this chapter.

What difference would it make if you incorporated these teachings, principles, and/or practices into your prayer life?

What questions, teachings, principles, and/or practices do you need to research and study further?

➢ **DIG DEEPER** into the following teachings, principles, and practices by prayerfully considering your responses, explanations, and descriptions. Record them in the space provided.

📖 **"I imagine Bildad thought he was speaking for God but it strikes me as funny that Job asked God a question and Bildad answered."** (p. 98)
Sometimes when our questions are directed to God, a well-meaning family member or friend will step in and answer the question for us. We are all too often prone to listen to that person's answer rather than waiting for and seeking God's response.

Recall a time you have witnessed someone direct a question to God, only to have a well-meaning family member or friend step in and answer that question.

What is the appropriate biblical response to such a situation?

📖 **"He (Job) knew that God was all powerful and sovereign and could do whatever He pleased, yet Job also knew that God was his only hope."** (p. 99)
Relate a situation when you recognized that God was your only hope.

Relate a situation when you did not recognize that God was your only hope.

Describe the difference in the outcomes of each situation.

📖 "(Job) **Chapter 18 has Job's friends harassing him again. This was ironic considering that their original purpose in coming to Job was to comfort him.**" (p.101)
Have there been times when friends who were supposed to be comforting you harassed you? Give an account of one such situation.

Have there been times when you should have been comforting someone but you actually harassed them instead? Give an account of one such situation.

   📖 **"And there it is again—Job's unshakable faith in a marvelous God. Even as Job accurately claimed that his entire calamity was from God, not because he had sinned, but because God had sovereignly chosen to allow calamity to fall on him, yet he took comfort in the knowledge that his God lives, and he will see Him someday."** (p.102)

Do you have a difficult time thinking that God sends calamity into your life? Explain why or why not?

How does your level of faith affect your ability to accept the calamity God sends into your life?

   📖 **"Job was a godly man, in whom God took pleasure … Yet, even a man such as this still had some lessons to learn."** (p.105)

What are some of the lessons Job still needed to learn about God?

Describe how your responses to situations indicate that you have or have not already learned the lessons you noted above.

Take time now to research and further study the questions, teachings, principles, and/or practices you recorded in the "Read" section of this chapter's study guide. Use your Bible, commentaries, and other resources (print or online) to study these questions, teachings, principles, and/or practices. Make notes of your answers and what you have learned from your research and study.

> **SCRIPTURE EMPHASIS**
> Carefully read and meditate upon Job 1:13-22. Reread the discussion of this passage on pages 97-98 in *Prayer: It's Not About You.* Write your answers to the following in the space provided.

What impact does your understanding of the following truths have in your prayer life?

◆ God is sovereign!

- ◆ Everything you have is from God.

- ◆ God's character never changes! God's character is not contingent upon my circumstances!

What questions do you have about this passage that are not addressed in the book?

Use your Bible, commentaries, and other resources (print or online) to find biblical answers for your questions, and record them below.

➤ **QUESTIONS FOR REFLECTION**
Prayerfully consider your answers, thoughts, and emotions. Record them in the space provided.

📖 What does the first chapter of Job teach us about Satan's power to harm us?

📖 What does Job say that helps us know he petitioned God with an open hand, ready to accept God's will regardless of how it affected him?

📖 Throughout most of the book, Job defends himself, claiming to have done no wrong. This claim was true. But toward the end of the book, Job repents. If he had done no wrong, what was Job repenting of?

📖 What often overlooked lesson about prayer can be found in the timing of God's restoration of Job?

➤ **NOW WHAT?**
Based on your study of the "Job" chapter, what specific teachings, principles, and/or practices do you need to incorporate into your prayer life? Record them below.

➤ **APPLY WHAT YOU LEARNED** by asking the Lord to strengthen your resolve to wait for His answers to your prayers. Pray that your knowledge and understanding of God would increase to a point where you recognize your only hope—in every situation—is God. Pray that you would be the type of friend who comforts others as you point them to Jesus (Hebrews 12:1-2). Ask Him to enable you to incorporate into your prayer life the teachings, principles, and/or practices you recorded earlier in the "Now What?" section of this chapter's study guide. Make notes of specific things for which you should pray.

➢ **MORE ANSWERS, NOTES, THOUGHTS, AND QUESTIONS**

NEW TESTAMENT

📖 *"When we come to God*
we are approaching
the throne of grace,
not the throne of merit."

Mark Janke

Pastor of Franklin Street Church, Louisville, Kentucky

CHAPTER 7: PRAYER IN THE NEW TESTAMENT

➤ **PRAY,** asking the Lord to open the eyes of your heart to learn what you need to know about prayer and that you would be sensitive to the Holy Spirit's conviction of sin, prompting you toward change. As the Holy Spirit convicts you of sin in your life, stop and ask forgiveness for that sin and for strength to choose not to continue practicing that sin.

➤ **READ** Chapter 7: "Prayer in the New Testament" in *Prayer: It's Not About You.*

List at least two of the teachings, principles, and/or practices that stood out to you as you read this chapter.

What difference would it make if you incorporated these teachings, principles, and/or practices into your prayer life?

What questions, teachings, principles, and/or practices do you need to research and study further?

➤ **DIG DEEPER** into the following teachings, principles, and practices by prayerfully considering your responses, explanations, and descriptions. Record them in the space provided.

📖 **"The New Testament teaches us that prayer is addressed …**

_____the Father,

_____the Son (or in the name of Jesus),

_____the help of the Holy Spirit (in the Spirit)."
(p. 111)

📖 **"The principle that we should address our prayers to God, the Father, has already been well established through Old Testament examples."** (p. 112)
Why do we address our prayers to God, the Father?

What are some New Testament passages that reinforce this principle?

📖 **"… the proper way to approach the Father is *through* the Son, or in the name of the Son."** (p. 113)
Why do we approach the Father through the Son, Jesus Christ?

Read Romans 8:33-35. Summarize this passage.

Find and list other passages that address the same issue as this Romans 8 passage.

In what ways does this passage encourage you to approach the Father through the Son, or in the name of the Son?

📖 **"One must remember though, this awesome and powerful resource** (the Holy Spirit) **available to us as we pray is only available** *if we actually take the time to pray!"* (p. 115)

Why is the power of the Holy Spirit important in prayer?

Tell of a time when you prayed about a situation, and did not worry.

Tell of a time when you did not pray about a situation, but worried instead.

Thinking about when you worried instead of prayed, describe the difference in that situation and the one when you prayed and the Holy Spirit strengthened you.

📖 **"Now, if I tell someone I will be praying for him or her, I write it down in my prayer journal so I remember it when I am praying."** (p. 116)
By what means do you remind yourself to pray about specific requests?

Take time now to research and further study the questions, teachings, principles, and/or practices you recorded in the "Read" section of this chapter's study guide. Use your Bible, commentaries, and other resources (print or online) to study these questions, teachings, principles, and/or practices. Make notes of your answers and what you have learned from your research and study.

➤ **SCRIPTURE EMPHASIS**
Carefully read and meditate upon John 12:27-28. Write your answers to the following in the space provided.

When were you in the midst of trouble and continually asked God to remove the trouble or save you?

When were you in the midst of trouble and continually asked God to strengthen you?

What questions do you have about this passage that are not addressed in the book?

Use your Bible, commentaries, and other resources (print or online) to find biblical answers for your questions, and record them below.

➤ **QUESTIONS FOR REFLECTION**
Prayerfully consider your answers, thoughts, and emotions. Record them in the space provided.

📖 **What is the basic role of the Father in regard to prayer?**

What is the basic role of the Son in regard to prayer?

What is the basic role of the Holy Spirit in regard to prayer?

➤ **NOW WHAT?**

Based on your study of the "Prayer in the New Testament" chapter, what specific teachings, principles, and/or practices do you need to incorporate into your prayer life? Record them below.

➤ **APPLY WHAT YOU LEARNED** by asking the Lord to enable you to study and better understand the Trinity (Father, Son, Holy Spirit) so that you have a better understanding of the role of each part of the Trinity in your prayers. Thank the Lord for the teachings, principles, and practices that you have learned. Ask Him to enable you to incorporate into your prayer life the teachings, principles, and/or practices you recorded earlier in the "Now What?" section of this chapter's study guide. Make notes of specific things for which you should pray.

➢ **MORE ANSWERS, NOTES, THOUGHTS, AND QUESTIONS**

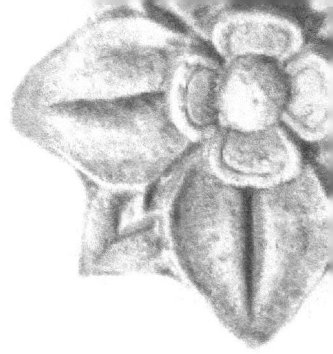

CHAPTER 8: TEACHINGS ON PRAYER

➤ **PRAY,** asking the Lord to open the eyes of your heart to learn what you need to know about prayer and that you would be sensitive to the Holy Spirit's conviction of sin, prompting you toward change. As the Holy Spirit convicts you of sin in your life, stop and ask forgiveness for that sin and for strength to choose not to continue practicing that sin.

➤ **READ** Chapter 8: "Teachings on Prayer" in *Prayer: It's Not About You.*

List at least two of the teachings, principles, and/or practices that stood out to you as you read this chapter.

What difference would it make if you incorporated these teachings, principles, and/or practices into your prayer life?

What questions, teachings, principles, and/or practices do you need to research and study further?

➤ **DIG DEEPER** into the following teachings, principles, and practices by prayerfully considering your responses, explanations, and descriptions. Record them in the space provided.

📖 **"Real love for others can only come about when we see what wretched sinners we ourselves truly are, thereby attaining a greater understanding of the depth of God's love for us."** (p. 120)
How does seeing what wretched sinners we are help us attain a greater understanding of the depth of God's love for us?

📖 **"Just as work requires the people working keep up their skills in order to continue being effective at their job, prayer requires that the person praying keep up his or her personal walk with God in order to continue praying effectively."** (p. 123)
How do you ensure you have a close personal walk with God?

Take time now to research and further study the questions, teachings, principles, and/or practices you recorded in the "Read" section of this chapter's study guide. Use your Bible, commentaries, and other resources (print or online) to study these questions, teachings, principles, and/or practices. Make notes of your answers and what you have learned from your research and study.

> **SCRIPTURE EMPHASIS**

Carefully read and meditate upon Mark 11:20-24. Write your answers to the following in the space provided.

What is the difference in basing your prayers on your faith in faith, as opposed to your faith in God?

What application does this passage have for your prayer life?

What questions do you have about this passage that are not addressed in the book?

Use your Bible, commentaries, and other resources (print or online) to find biblical answers for your questions, and record them below.

➤ **QUESTIONS FOR REFLECTION**

Prayerfully consider your answers, thoughts, and emotions. Record them in the space provided.

📖 Renowned author D. A. Carson writes, "If we are to improve our prayers, we must strengthen our loving." According to Luke 7, how do we accomplish this goal?

📖 Love for others is a natural by-product of what?

📖 How does Jesus explain this truth in Luke 7:47?

📖 List three ways in which prayer is like work.

📖 **Finish this quote by Elisabeth Elliot:**

"Prayer is no game _____ _____ _____

_____ _____ _____.

It is something to be engaged in, not _____ _____."

📖 **The Scriptures primarily make two points regarding what enhances and what detracts from our prayers. What are these two points?**

📖 **Break it down a bit more: Personal holiness (our personal walk with God through reading and observing His Word, spending time with Him in prayer and worship, etc.), or the lack thereof, reflects what?**

📖 **Godly living or the lack thereof reflects what?**

📖 **Is fasting mandatory? Why then do we fast?**

📖 **What should be the focus of our faith when we pray?**

📖 **If we truly have faith when we pray, does that mean we will always get what we ask for in prayer?**

➤ NOW WHAT?

Based on your study of the "Teachings on Prayer" chapter, what specific teachings, principles, and/or practices do you need to incorporate into your prayer life? Record them below.

➤ **APPLY WHAT YOU LEARNED** by asking the Lord to enable you to recognize and better understand the depth of His love for you. Pray that you will become more aware of the wretchedness of your sin and be quick to seek forgiveness and repent. Ask Him to enable you to be an effective prayer warrior. Ask Him to enable you to incorporate into your prayer life the teachings, principles, and/or practices you recorded earlier in the "Now What?" section of this chapter's study guide. Make notes of specific things for which you should pray.

➤ **MORE ANSWERS, NOTES, THOUGHTS, AND QUESTIONS**

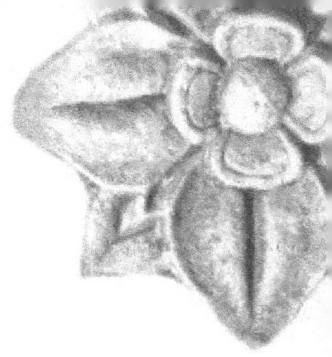

CHAPTER 9: MORE TEACHINGS ON PRAYER

➢ **PRAY,** asking the Lord to open the eyes of your heart to learn what you need to know about prayer and that you would be sensitive to the Holy Spirit's conviction of sin, prompting you toward change. As the Holy Spirit convicts you of sin in your life, stop and ask forgiveness for that sin and for strength to choose not to continue practicing that sin.

➢ **READ** Chapter 9: "More Teachings on Prayer" in *Prayer: It's Not About You.*

List at least two of the teachings, principles, and/or practices that stood out to you as you read this chapter.

What difference would it make if you incorporated these teachings, principles, and/or practices into your prayer life?

What questions, teachings, principles, and/or practices do you need to research and study further?

➢ **DIG DEEPER** into the following teachings, principles, and practices by prayerfully considering your responses, explanations, and descriptions. Record them in the space provided.

📖 **"… what about praise when we are hurting and pouring our hearts out to God?"** (p. 139)
Use Philippians 4:4-9 to explain how you can give praise and thanksgiving when you are hurting.

What is the result of faithful dependence on Christ and a consistent Christ-focused prayer life?

📖 **"David made it clear that praise is a choice and an important part of communing with God regardless of circumstances."** (p. 139)
In Psalm 69 what is the context in which David gives praise to God?

Recount the context in which Job proclaimed, "Shall we accept good from God, and not trouble?" (Job 2:10) How was it possible for Job to respond to his situation in this manner?

List several things that should make up the content of our prayers.

📖 **"What a marvelous condition in which to find a person or to be in ourselves—clothed, in our right mind, and sitting at the feet of Jesus."** (p. 144)
How does an encounter with Jesus through prayer and reading the Bible bring about clarity in our thinking and a desire to walk more closely with Him?

📖 **"First Thessalonians 5:17 tells us to pray continually."** (p. 146)
What does it mean to pray continually? Include an example of what praying continually does not mean.

Take time now to research and further study the questions, teachings, principles, and/or practices you recorded in the "Read" section of this chapter's study guide. Use your Bible, commentaries, and other resources (print or online) to study these questions, teachings, principles, and/or practices. Make notes of your answers and what you have learned from your research and study.

➢ **SCRIPTURE EMPHASIS**
Carefully read and meditate upon Acts 12:12-16. Write your answers to the following in the space provided.

Describe a time when you have fervently prayed for something to happen, and then been amazed when your prayer was answered in the way you wanted it to be answered.

What causes you to not believe God will answer your prayers in the way you want them answered?

What questions do you have about this passage that are not addressed in the book?

Use your Bible, commentaries, and other resources (print or online) to find biblical answers for your questions, and record them below.

➢ **QUESTIONS FOR REFLECTION**
Prayerfully consider your answers, thoughts, and emotions. Record them in the space provided.

📖 **Should praise and thanksgiving be offered to God even in sad or difficult circumstances?** Explain why or why not.

📖 As a means of review, list (again) some of the elements that should be included in our prayers. (This is a review of the "David / the Psalms" chapter beginning on page 31.)

📖 What does the word supplication mean?

📖 What are some synonyms for supplication?

📖 In the last part of this section, Harriet told the story of the demon possessed man. What was his condition after the demon had been cast out of him? (Hint: It is a condition that we would all do well to be in and one that Harriet often recites in her prayers as a condition into which she asks God to put her and others in.)

📖 **List some possible reasons why our prayers are not always answered immediately.**

➤ **NOW WHAT?**

Based on your study of the "More Teachings on Prayer" chapter, what specific teachings, principles, and/or practices do you need to incorporate into your prayer life? Record them below.

➤ **APPLY WHAT YOU LEARNED** by asking the Lord to enable you to learn more about Him so that your faith increases, thus allowing you to pray trusting that He will answer your prayer according to His will. Pray the Lord would increase your desire to know Him better. Pray He would teach you to pray continually. Ask Him to enable you to incorporate into your prayer life the teachings, principles, and/or practices you recorded earlier in the "Now What?" section of this chapter's study guide. Make notes of specific things for which you should pray.

➢ **MORE ANSWERS, NOTES, THOUGHTS, AND QUESTIONS**

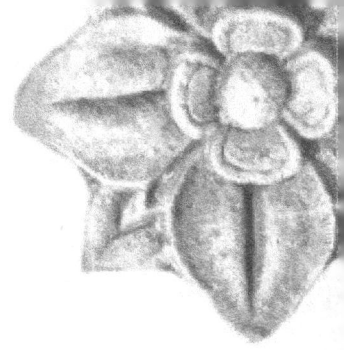

CHAPTER 10: JESUS

➢ **PRAY,** asking the Lord to open the eyes of your heart to learn what you
need to know about prayer and that you would be sensitive to the Holy
Spirit's conviction of sin, prompting you toward change. As the Holy
Spirit convicts you of sin in your life, stop and ask forgiveness for that sin
and for strength to choose not to continue practicing that sin.

➢ **READ** Chapter 10: "Jesus" in *Prayer: It's Not About You*.

List at least two of the teachings, principles, and/or practices that stood out to you
as you read this chapter.

What difference would it make if you incorporated these teachings, principles,
and/or practices into your prayer life?

What questions, teachings, principles, and/or practices do you need to research and
study further?

➢ **DIG DEEPER** into the following teachings, principles, and practices by prayerfully considering your responses, explanations, and descriptions. Record them in the space provided.

📖 **"The act of praying privately is itself an act of faith."** (pp. 152-153)
Explain how the act of praying privately is an act of faith.

📖 **"Charles Haddon Spurgeon once wrote 'That God predestines, and yet that man is responsible, are two facts that few can see clearly ….'"** (p. 157)
How does a Christ-follower reconcile these two seemingly contradictory truths?

📖 **"… we should remember what I John 4:4 tells us—that the One who is in us, referring to the Holy Spirit who was given to all believers, is greater than the one who is in the world."** (p. 159-160)
By what process do Christ-followers get into situations where they think and act as though they are not able to overcome their own sin and/or the evil one?

📖 **"Prayer was an active part of Jesus' life. It was routine to Him rather than occasional."** (p. 161)

In what ways is praying an active part of your life?

What can you do to make praying a more active part of your life?

How can you guard against your prayers becoming monotonous and self-serving?

📖 **"Jesus made it clear in these verses that sometimes when we pray publicly our prayers are a witness to those around us."** (p. 163)

In what circumstances would your public prayer witness to those around you?

Describe how public prayer can be sinful. Give specific examples.

Take time now to research and further study the questions, teachings, principles, and/or practices you recorded in the "Read" section of this chapter's study guide. Use your Bible, commentaries, and other resources (print or online) to study these questions, teachings, principles, and/or practices. Make notes of your answers and what you have learned from your research and study.

➢ **SCRIPTURE EMPHASIS**
Carefully read and meditate upon Romans 9:11-15. Write your answers to the following in the space provided.

Tell about a situation in your life, or one you have witnessed, where God has thwarted man's plan. You may use biblical examples also.

Carefully read and meditate upon Acts 5:38-39. Write your answers to the following in the space provided.

According to this passage, how do we know if a plan is of God or man?

What questions do you have about these two passages that are not addressed in the book?

Use your Bible, commentaries, and other resources (print or online) to find biblical answers for your questions, and record them below.

> ➤ **QUESTIONS FOR REFLECTION**
> Prayerfully consider your answers, thoughts, and emotions. Record them in the space provided.

📖 **What did Jesus mean by His instruction not to recite meaningless words when we pray, like the Gentiles did?**

📖 **In Matthew 6:6, Jesus says to go into a room, shut the door, and pray in secret. Yet, at the same time, He models public prayer. Are these contradictions?** Explain why or why not.

📖 **What is a caution regarding public prayer?**

📖 **Why was Jesus sorrowful even to death at the Garden of Gethsemane? What loomed before Him there?**

📖 **What did Jesus pray in this moment of agony?**

📖 **What two amazing traits and behaviors, which we should imitate, did Jesus display on Calvary?**

➢ **NOW WHAT?**

Based on your study of the "Jesus" chapter, what specific teachings, principles, and/or practices do you need to incorporate into your prayer life? Record them below.

➢ **APPLY WHAT YOU LEARNED** by asking the Lord to strengthen you to boldly live out your faith through your private and public prayers. Pray that the Lord would increase your ability to believe, in faith, the truths about God and His work that you cannot reconcile in your mind. Pray that the Lord would enable you to live your life in such a way that you are always cognizant of the fact that the indwelling Holy Spirit is greater than the evil one or any worldly force that comes against you. Ask Him to enable you to incorporate into your prayer life the teachings, principles, and/or practices you recorded earlier in the "Now What?" section of this chapter's study guide. Make notes of specific things for which you should pray.

➤ **MORE ANSWERS, NOTES, THOUGHTS, AND QUESTIONS**

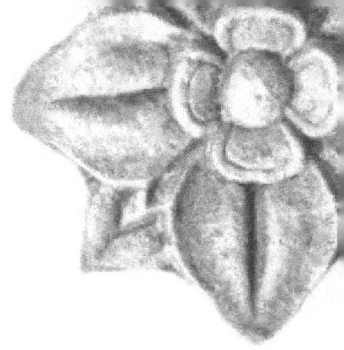

CHAPTER 11: PAUL

➤ **PRAY,** asking the Lord to open the eyes of your heart to learn what you need to know about prayer and that you would be sensitive to the Holy Spirit's conviction of sin, prompting you toward change. As the Holy Spirit convicts you of sin in your life, stop and ask forgiveness for that sin and for strength to choose not to continue practicing that sin.

➤ **READ** Chapter 11: "Paul" in *Prayer: It's Not About You.*

List at least two of the teachings, principles, and/or practices that stood out to you as you read this chapter.

What difference would it make if you incorporated these teachings, principles, and/or practices into your prayer life?

What questions, teachings, principles, and/or practices do you need to research and study further?

➢ **DIG DEEPER** into the following teachings, principles, and practices by prayerfully considering your responses, explanations, and descriptions. Record them in the space provided.

📖 **"We should earnestly pray about eternal issues as Paul did, but not at the neglect of the physical ones. Remember Jesus himself taught us to ask for our daily bread when we pray."** (p. 182)
How can Christ-followers ensure that their prayers are not unbalanced (e.g. all prayers pertain to physical needs)?

📖 **"Other than giving thanks and aligning with God's will, what were the specific things on Paul's heart when he prayed?"** (p. 185)
Give examples from Scripture of specific things that were on Paul's heart when he prayed.

Read Acts 28:8-9. How you would explain to a new Christ-follower the principle of prayer Paul demonstrates in these verses?

📖 **"Paul often asked others to pray for him, too."** (p. 186)
How does your sin of pride stop you from asking others to pray for you?

From the section "Paul's Teachings" (p. 187), explain why we need to incorporate Paul's various instructions about prayer into our prayer lives.

From the section "Live Peacefully" (p. 188), describe how your prayer life affects your ability to live peacefully with others.

📖 **"Sometimes more than one teaching can be found in the same verse."** (p. 187)
For each of the teachings below, find and list Scripture passages that reinforce the teaching. Find at least three passages that are not found in the book.

📖 **"Joy and Thanksgiving"** (pp. 187-188)

📖 **"Perseverance"** (p. 188)

📖 **"Live Peacefully"** (p. 188)

Take time now to research and further study the questions, teachings, principles, and/or practices you recorded in the "Read" section of this chapter's study guide. Use your Bible, commentaries, and other resources (print or online) to study these questions, teachings, principles, and/or practices. Make notes of your answers and what you have learned from your research and study.

➤ **SCRIPTURE EMPHASIS**

Carefully read and meditate upon Acts 9:26-30. Write your answers to the following in the space provided.

What did Barnabas do for the Apostle Paul (formerly Saul) when he came to Jerusalem to join the disciples who were afraid of Paul?

Carefully read and meditate upon Acts 11:25-26. Write your answers to the following in the space provided.

What does Barnabas demonstrate for us in his relationship with Paul during the year they were together? What do we call that today?

What questions do you have about these two passages that are not addressed in the book?

Use your Bible, commentaries, and other resources (print or online) to find biblical answers for your questions, and record them below.

> ➢ **QUESTIONS FOR REFLECTION**
Prayerfully consider your answers, thoughts, and emotions. Record them in the space provided.

📖 **What is the usual focus of Paul's prayers?**

📖 **Is Paul's focus a better way to pray?**

📖 **What was especially unique about Paul's encounter with Jesus?**

22

➤ **NOW WHAT?**

Based on your study of the "Paul" chapter, what specific teachings, principles, and/or practices do you need to incorporate into your prayer life? Record them below.

➤ **APPLY WHAT YOU LEARNED** by asking the Lord to strengthen you to give thanks in whatever circumstance you find yourself, and that you will be eager to align your will with God's will. Pray the Lord would enable you to develop a more fruitful prayer life. Ask Him to enable you to incorporate into your prayer life the teachings, principles, and/or practices you recorded earlier in the "Now What?" section of this chapter's study guide. Make notes of specific things for which you should pray.

➤ **MORE ANSWERS, NOTES, THOUGHTS, AND QUESTIONS**

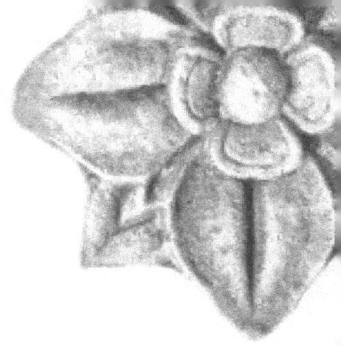

Chapter 12: Other Prayers in the New Testament

> **Pray,** asking the Lord to open the eyes of your heart to learn what you need to know about prayer and that you would be sensitive to the Holy Spirit's conviction of sin, prompting you toward change. As the Holy Spirit convicts you of sin in your life, stop and ask forgiveness for that sin and for strength to choose not to continue practicing that sin.

> **Read** Chapter 12: "Other Prayers in the New Testament" in *Prayer: It's Not About You.*

List at least two of the teachings, principles, and/or practices that stood out to you as you read this chapter.

What difference would it make if you incorporated these teachings, principles, and/or practices into your prayer life?

What questions, teachings, principles, and/or practices do you need to research and study further?

➤ **DIG DEEPER** into the following teachings, principles, and practices by prayerfully considering your responses, explanations, and descriptions. Record them in the space provided.

📖 **"From that day forward** (the day of Pentecost) **the Holy Spirit has been given to every believer at the time of their conversion and continues to indwell us until we die."** (p. 191)
How would you convey to a new Christ-follower the importance of the indwelling Holy Spirit in the life of a Christ-follower?

📖 **"This passage (Luke 1:13-17) is one of the clearest examples of God's two-pronged work to answer the heartfelt prayers of His people while simultaneously fulfilling His own divine purposes."** (p. 192)
Briefly explain this two-pronged work of God.

📖 **"This way of thinking is dangerous. It would have us picturing God as a less than all-powerful being who must have been pleasantly surprised ...."** (p. 193)
What way of thinking is dangerous? Explain why this way of thinking is dangerous.

📖 **"Zechariah and his wife Elizabeth were very old."** (p. 194) See Luke 1:6-7. Tell about a time when your faith in God was undermined by your perception of the facts of a situation (they were very old, etc.) so that you did not pray about that situation.

What did you learn about God during this time?

What did you learn about prayer during this time?

📖 **"In answering this** (Zechariah's) **prayer, God confirmed some of what Scripture teaches about God's nature and prayer."** (p. 195) What does God's answer to Zechariah's prayer teach us about God's nature and prayer?

📖 **"... God's presence was accompanied by ... and other bold signs."** (p. 196) For each Scripture reference below, list the signs that accompanied God's presence.

📖 Exodus 19:18

📖 Job 40:9

📖 Isaiah 29:6

Take time now to research and further study the questions, teachings, principles, and/or practices you recorded in the "Read" section of this chapter's study guide. Use your Bible, commentaries, and other resources (print or online) to study these questions, teachings, principles, and/or practices. Make notes of your answers and what you have learned from your research and study.

> **SCRIPTURE EMPHASIS**

Carefully read and meditate upon Luke 1:5-24. Write your answers to the following in the space provided.

List the biblical principles included in this passage.

How can these same principles be applied to your prayer life and Christian walk?

What questions do you have about this passage that are not addressed in the book?

Use your Bible, commentaries, and other resources (print or online) to find biblical answers for your questions, and record them below.

➤ **QUESTIONS FOR REFLECTION**

Prayerfully consider your answers, thoughts, and emotions. Record them in the space provided.

📖 **What is the basic difference in the way prayers are recorded in the Old Testament as opposed to the New Testament?**

📖 **What two new insights do we gain from Zechariah's prayer for a child?**

📖 **What truth about prayer is vividly portrayed in the book of Revelation?**

➢ **NOW WHAT?**

Based on your study of the "Other Prayers in the New Testament" chapter, what specific teachings, principles, and/or practices do you need to incorporate into your prayer life? Record them below.

➢ **APPLY WHAT YOU LEARNED** by asking the Lord to give you a passion to know Him better so that you more fully understand WHO He is (His character). Pray you would learn to trust God's sovereignty, even if you do not understand how God is 100% sovereign and we are 100% responsible for the choices we make and to pray. Ask Him to enable you to incorporate into your prayer life the teachings, principles, and/or practices you recorded earlier in the "Now What?" section of this chapter's study guide. Make notes of specific things for which you should pray.

➢ **MORE ANSWERS, NOTES, THOUGHTS, AND QUESTIONS**

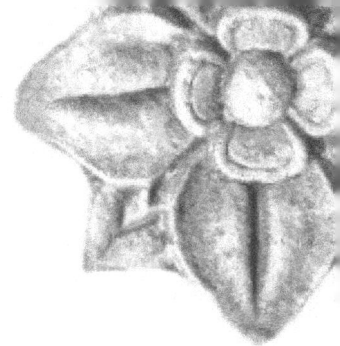

CHAPTER 13: THE AWESOME POWER OF PRAYER

➢ **PRAY,** asking the Lord to open the eyes of your heart to learn what you need to know about prayer and that you would be sensitive to the Holy Spirit's conviction of sin, prompting you toward change. As the Holy Spirit convicts you of sin in your life, stop and ask forgiveness for that sin and for strength to choose not to continue practicing that sin.

➢ **READ** Chapter 13: "The Awesome Power of Prayer" in *Prayer: It's Not About You*.

List at least two of the teachings, principles, and/or practices that stood out to you as you read this chapter.

What difference would it make if you incorporated these teachings, principles, and/or practices into your prayer life?

What questions, teachings, principles, and/or practices do you need to research and study further?

➢ **DIG DEEPER** into the following teachings, principles, and practices by prayerfully considering your responses, explanations, and descriptions. Record them in the space provided.

On pages 199-203 in *Prayer: It's Not About You*, review the occurrences in the Bible that came either right after, or simultaneously, with prayer.

Read each passage below and name the biblical principle of prayer that you find.

Exodus 14:15-21

Judges 16:26-31

I Kings 18:36-38

II Kings 4:32-34

II Kings 19:35

Esther 4:16

Job 42:10

Isaiah 38:8

Mark 6:46-49

Mark 9:29

John 11:41-44

Acts 4:31

Acts 9:11

Acts 10:1-8

Acts 12:5-10

Revelation 1:10

Take time now to research and further study the questions, teachings, principles, and/or practices you recorded in the "Read" section of this chapter's study guide. Use your Bible, commentaries, and other resources (print or online) to study these questions, teachings, principles, and/or practices. Make notes of your answers and what you have learned from your research and study.

> **SCRIPTURE EMPHASIS**

Carefully read and meditate upon Luke 22:39–23:56. Write your answers to the following in the space provided.

List the biblical principles included in this passage.

How can you incorporate these biblical principles into your prayer life?

What questions do you have about this passage that are not addressed in the book?

Use your Bible, commentaries, and other resources (print or online) to find biblical answers for your questions, and record them below.

➢ **QUESTIONS FOR REFLECTION**
Prayerfully consider your answers, thoughts, and emotions. Record them in the space provided.

As you consider the examples given in this chapter, consider and list what these prayer warriors have in common.

Give at least two examples of when you have personally experienced the awesome power of prayer.

Describe your responses to the experiences you listed earlier.

➢ **NOW WHAT?**

Based on your study of the "The Awesome Power of Prayer" chapter, what specific teachings, principles, and/or practices do you need to incorporate into your prayer life? Record them below.

➢ **APPLY WHAT YOU LEARNED** by asking the Lord to ignite your passion for prayer and knowing Him better. Ask Him to increase your faith. Pray that as you incorporate into your prayer life the teachings, principles, and practices you have been studying in this book, that you would understand and experience the awesome power of prayer. Ask Him to enable you to incorporate into your prayer life the teachings, principles, and/or practices you recorded earlier in the "Now What?" section of this chapter's study guide. Make notes of specific things for which you should pray.

➤ **MORE ANSWERS, NOTES, THOUGHTS, AND QUESTIONS**

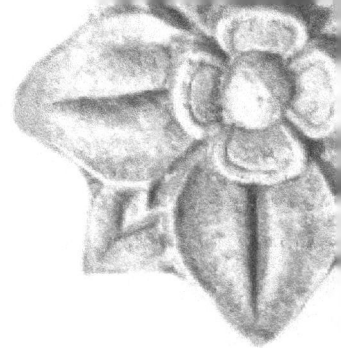

CHAPTER 14: CONCLUSION

➤ **PRAY,** asking the Lord to open the eyes of your heart to learn what you need to know about prayer and that you would be sensitive to the Holy Spirit's conviction of sin, prompting you toward change. As the Holy Spirit convicts you of sin in your life, stop and ask forgiveness for that sin and for strength to choose not to continue practicing that sin.

➤ **READ** Chapter 14: "Conclusion" in *Prayer: It's Not About You.*

List at least two of the teachings, principles, and/or practices that stood out to you as you read this chapter.

What difference would it make if you incorporated these teachings, principles, and/or practices into your prayer life?

What questions, teachings, principles, and/or practices do you need to research and study further?

➤ **DIG DEEPER** into the following teachings, principles, and practices by prayerfully considering your responses, explanations, and descriptions. Record them in the space provided.

Page 208 lists ten themes or points of prayer from Chapter 3: "David / the Psalms." Review these in Chapter 3: "David / the Psalms" on pages 38–60 of *Prayer: It's Not About You.*

Why do you need to, and how will you, incorporate each of these themes into your prayer life?

📖 1) **Our prayers should be made to God the Father through the Son at the prompting and with the help of the Holy Spirit.**

📖 2) **Prayers are filled with praise and thanksgiving.**

📖 3) **We come humbly to God, confessing our sins, asking for forgiveness, and recognizing our personal unworthiness before God.**

📖 **4) We can petition God based on His character.**

📖 **God's steadfast love**

📖 **Faithfulness**

📖 **Fortress / Stronghold / Rock / Refuge**

📖 **Shield**

📖 **Help**

📖 **Deliverer / Redeemer**

📖 **Goodness and Mercy**

📖 **Graciousness**

📖 **Righteous / Upright / Holy**

📖 **Other Character Traits**

📖 **5) We can petition God based on His promises.**

📖 **6) We can petition God based His ability to answer our prayers.**

📖 **7) We can petition God based on His will.**

📖 **8) We can petition God based on His glory.**

📖 9) We should recognize what He has done in our lives.

📖 10) We can pour out our hearts to Him.

📖 "Like a good lawyer arguing before a judge, when we come before God in our prayers, we too can stand on the law and precedents." (p. 212)
How would you explain to a new Christ-follower what it means to stand on the law and the precedents?

Take time now to research and further study the questions, teachings, principles, and/or practices you recorded in the "Read" section of this chapter's study guide. Use your Bible, commentaries, and other resources (print or online) to study these questions, teachings, principles, and/or practices. Make notes of your answers and what you have learned from your research and study.

➢ **SCRIPTURE EMPHASIS**
Carefully read and meditate upon Isaiah 59:15-16. Write your answers to the following in the space provided.

Why is it important for us to intercede for others?

What application does this passage have for your prayer life?

What questions do you have about this passage that are not addressed in the book?

Use your Bible, commentaries, and other resources (print or online) to find biblical answers for your questions, and record them below.

➢ **QUESTIONS FOR REFLECTION**
Prayerfully consider your answers, thoughts, and emotions. Record them in the space provided.

In what ways can you become a more effective prayer warrior?

Explain the impact unconfessed sin has in the effectiveness of your prayers.

How does knowing and understanding God's character help you bring everything to Him in prayer?

Explain why prayer is about God—not you!

➤ **NOW WHAT?**

Based on your study of the "Conclusion" chapter, what specific teachings, principles, and/or practices do you need to incorporate into your prayer life? Record them below.

> ➤ **APPLY WHAT YOU LEARNED** by asking the Lord to ignite your passion for prayer and knowing Him better. Ask Him to help you incorporate the teachings, principles, and practices you reviewed in this chapter. Thank the Lord for the teachings, principles, and practices that you have learned. Ask Him to enable you to incorporate into your prayer life the teachings, principles, and/or practices you recorded earlier in the "Now What?" section of this chapter's study guide. Make notes of specific things for which you should pray.

➤ **MORE ANSWERS, NOTES, THOUGHTS, AND QUESTIONS**

WRAP UP

Review the teachings, principles, and/or practices in each chapter of the study guide that you have studied.

➢ **LIST** from each chapter of the study guide any teachings, principles, and/or practices of which you still do not have a good understanding. Also list questions that remain unanswered after your research and study.

➤ **LIST** (continued)

➤ **PERSIST** until you have researched and studied each teaching, principle, and/or practice from the "List" section, so that you have a good enough understanding of each one.

➢ **PERSIST** (continued)

➤ **ANSWER** the questions from the "List" and "Persist" sections as you would explain them to a new Christ-follower.

➤ **ANSWER** (continued)

EVEN MORE ANSWERS, NOTES, THOUGHTS, AND QUESTIONS

EVEN MORE ANSWERS, NOTES, THOUGHTS, AND QUESTIONS

FOR PRACTICE AND MORE STUDY

Now that you have completed this study of *Prayer: It's Not About You*, it is important that you continue to practice praying and studying prayer.

Practice

- ◆ Prayer Partner

  Find a committed Christ-following friend to be a prayer partner with whom you can share anything, who will be faithful to pray for you. Someone with whom you will be excited to share how God is answering your prayers.

- ◆ Prayer Journal (See "Sample Prayer Journal" on page 170 of this study guide.)

  We strongly encourage you to begin a Prayer Journal in which you can write:

  - ▪ the things about and for which you are praying,
  - ▪ your sin and the confession of that sin,
  - ▪ what the Lord is teaching you,
  - ▪ thoughts and feelings about what you are learning and experiencing,
  - ▪ anything else that comes to mind.

  Make certain that you leave room to go back and record how the Lord answered your prayers, and the things He taught you as you prayed and waited for answers. Take time to go back through your Prayer Journal regularly. Reflect upon the things the Lord has accomplished in and through your prayers and how your understanding of Him has grown.

  The form and format of your Prayer Journal is not important. You may use an inexpensive spiral-bound notepad or a bound journal in which you can write. Create Prayer Journal pages you type into your computer, or use Prayer Journal pages to print, 3-hole punch, and put in a 3-ring binder. We have included a "Sample Prayer Journal" on page 170 of this study guide. You can also find samples online by searching "Prayer Journal."

◆ Prayer App

Download a prayer app to organize your prayer requests and remind you to pray.

FOR FURTHER READING AND STUDY

Books about Prayer

A Call to Prayer – J. C. Ryle
A Call to Spiritual Reformation: Priorities from Paul and His Prayer – D. A. Carson
A Woman's Call to Prayer: Making Your Desire to Pray a Reality – Elizabeth George
Disciplines of a Godly Man – R. Kent Hughes
Hudson Taylor's Spiritual Secret – Dr. Hudson Taylor
Life and Diary of David Brainerd – Edited: Jonathan Edwards
Prayer: Experiencing Awe and Intimacy with God – Tim Keller
Praying Backwards – Bryan Chapell
Praying the Bible – Donald S. Whitney
Praying the Names of God – Ann Spangler
Reaching the Ear of God: Praying More and More Like Jesus – Wayne A. Mack
Spurgeon on Prayer – Charles Spurgeon
The Autobiography of George Muller – George Muller
The Complete Works of E. M. Bounds on Prayer – E. M. Bounds
The Heart of Prayer – Jerram Barrs
The Invisible War: What Every Believer Needs to Know About Satan – Chip Ingram
The Mighty Weakness of John Knox – Douglas Bond
The Praying Wife – Stormie O'Martian
With Christ in the School of Prayer – Andrew Murray
With the Master: On Our Knees – Susan J. Heck

Devotionals

A Shelter in the Time of Storm: Meditations on God and Trouble – Paul David Tripp
Cross Talking: A Daily Gospel for Transforming Addicts – Mark E. Shaw
Glimpses of the Savior – Shirley Crowder & Harriet E. Michael
My Utmost for His Highest – Oswald Chambers
New Morning Mercies: A Daily Gospel Devotional – Paul David Tripp
Through Baca's Valley – J. C. Philpot
Valley of Vision: A Collection of Puritan Prayers – Arthur G. Bennett
Whiter Than Snow: Meditations on Sin and Mercy – Paul David Tripp

SAMPLE PRAYER JOURNAL

Date: _____
My prayer:

_____

_____

_____

_____

Scripture/Bible Promises:

_____

_____

_____

Who is praying with me about this?

_____

_____

Date God answered my prayer: _____
How God answered my prayer:

_____

_____

_____

_____

What God taught me through the process of praying this prayer and waiting for His answer:

_____

_____

_____

With whom did I share how God answered this prayer?

_____

ABOUT THE AUTHOR

SHIRLEY CROWDER

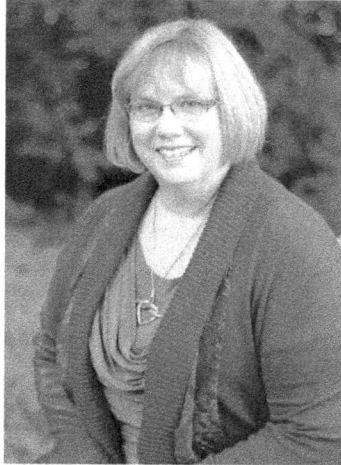

Born in a mission guest house under the shade of a mango tree in Nigeria, West Africa, where her parents served as missionaries, Shirley is passionate about disciple-making, which is conducted in and through myriad ministry opportunities.

She is a biblical counselor and co-host of "Think on These Things," a Birmingham, Alabama, radio/TV program for women. Shirley is commissioned by and serves on the national Advisory Team for The Addiction Connection. She co-authored the chapter, "Paul and Women in Ministry" in the book *Paul the Counselor* published by Focus Publishing; and has several articles which have appeared in *The Gadsden Times'* Faith section's Paper Pulpit. She and Harriet E. Michael are co-authors of a holiday devotional, *Glimpses of the Savior*, published by TMP Books in 2015.

Shirley has spiritual children, grandchildren, and great-grandchildren serving the Lord in various ministry and secular positions throughout the world.

Follow her on:
Blog: www.throughthelensofScripture.com
Facebook: www.facebook.com/shirleycrowder
Twitter: www.twitter.com/ShirleyJCrowder
Amazon: www.amazon.com/author/shirleycrowder

ALSO BY THE AUTHOR

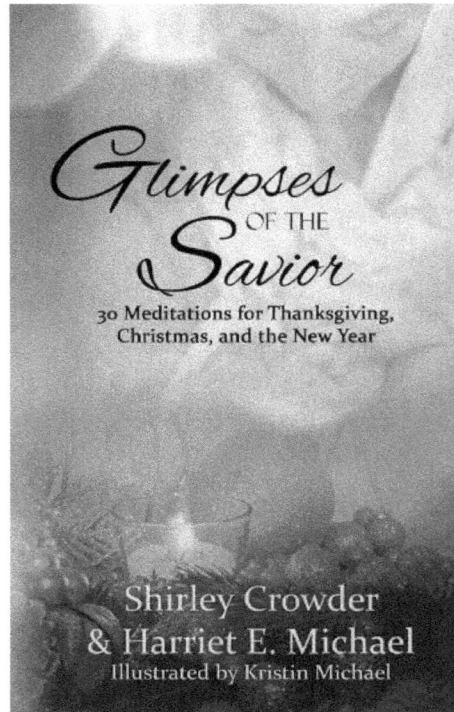

Finding Jesus Among the Celebrations and Decorations

In early November, we get busy preparing for Thanksgiving, Christmas, and the New Year, and we often forget the real meanings behind these celebrations.

We can guard against this by preparing our hearts to seek Him as we focus on God's Word and by remembering that Thanksgiving is a time to give God thanks; Christmas is the celebration of the Savior's birth; the New Year brings new beginnings. Then, as we go about doing the things the Lord has called us to do where He has called us to do them, we catch Glimpses of the Savior and biblical truth in the things we experience and observe.

These devotionals are based on memories of Thanksgiving, Christmas, and New Year Celebrations in Africa and America. May the Holy Spirit work through these meditations to help readers recognize Glimpses of the Savior in the things they observe, and become skilled at finding Jesus among the celebrations and decorations.

**Available on Kindle and in paperback from Amazon
and most bookstores by request.**

RECENTLY RELEASED BY PIX-N-PENS PUBLISHING

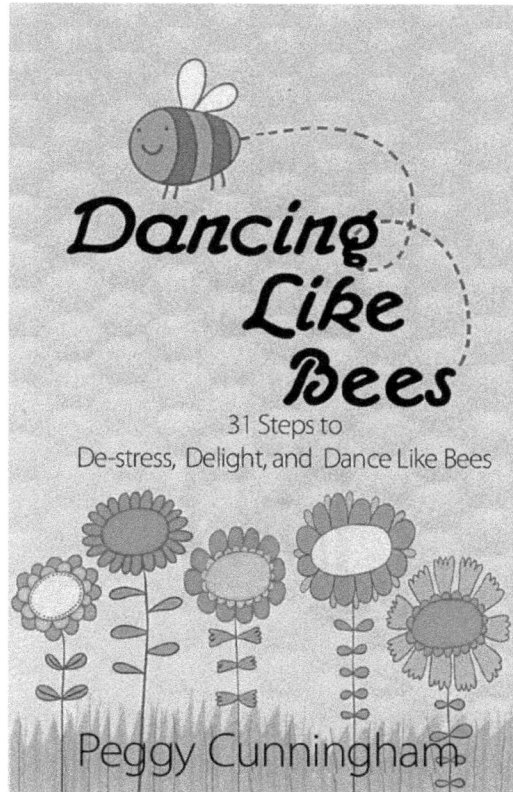

Dancing Like Bees
31 Steps to De-stress, Delight, and Dance Like Bees

Through the thirty-one devotions, this book examines what Peggy learned about God's intricate creation of the honeybee and how it speaks direction into our need for living peaceful, productive lives while overcoming stress and achieving joy. God is faithful always, and His creation magnifies His majesty if we take time to seek Him in everyday situations—even through the honeybee.

**Thank you
for reading our books!**

**Look for other books
published by**

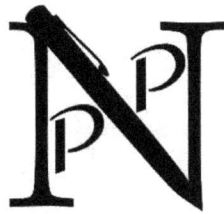

Pix-N-Pens Publishing
An imprint of Write Integrity Press
www.WriteIntegrity.com

www.ingramcontent.com/pod-product-compliance
Lightning Source LLC
Chambersburg PA
CBHW080049280326
41934CB00014B/3263